Is Big Pharma Behind The Ban on Kratom?

By Simon Luria

I0447532

Copyright information

Luria, Simon

Is Big Pharma Behind The Ban on Kratom?

—1st ed

Printed in the United States of America

Cover images : #64844291

Open hand raised, Stop Kratom Addiction sign painted © ijacky

Book Cover Design: Simon Luria

Introduction

The United States is in the midst of the worst Opioid and Heroin epidemic in history. Never have we seen so many people perish due to overdoses of these substances. So many senseless deaths, deaths that can be readily avoided.

Modern medicine today has very little to offer those who are hopelessly addicted to Opioids and Heroin. What they do provide is either detoxing agents or weak substitutes in order to stave off the horrendous withdrawal sickness individuals who take opioids and Heroin experience when they do not have the ability to obtain their respective substances. In many ways, the inadequacy of modern medicine to address these issues is for the most part, due to the "War on Drugs." Addiction at least as far as law enforcement is concerned is not considered a health issue but a social and moral one, and thus they are ill-prepared to address it in the way that they should.

Some addicts know they are in deep trouble and have sought professional help, but the "professionals" have let them down. Due to the ineffectiveness of the addiction treatment juggernaut, the addicted person goes out to seek some kind of alternative that will allow them to eventually stop drugs without experiencing serious withdrawal. One of these alternatives is called Kratom. Kratom is a plant that has been shown to have a very profound effect upon the lives of those addicted to opioids and Heroin, in fact, it is a lifesaver for many. At least, it was until the DEA recently banned it and made it a controlled substance. Once so readily available, is now illegal to possess. The question remains, why did they ban it? It was shown to be very useful to those who were trying to kick their dependence on Heroin and opioids. In fact, it was too effective. Are there risks to taking Kratom? Of course, just like with every medicine or alternative remedy, but the overall risk is low compared to its proven benefits.

 In this book, I am going to explore what Kratom is and why I believe the DEA banned it. I will present information that will illustrate that the only real reason the DEA banned Kratom was because Big Pharma aka the pharmaceutical companies want Kratom to themselves because they know it works. In fact, they have known about its properties for quite some time now. They have no interest in its sale right now since it will cut into the Opioid Pill market which is at the time of this writing, the largest of all pharmaceutical markets. They have in a sense, effectively bribed the government to take something that gave hope to thousands and made it into a money-making machine, a machine that has always been known for its ruthlessness.

What Is Kratom?

Kratom is a very interesting plant, unlike other herbs that are readily available; this one has a truly palpable effect upon the brain and body.

The Scientific name for Kratom is *Mitragyna speciosa; it* is an evergreen tree that thrives in tropical climates. Interestingly enough, it is in the coffee family of trees, Rubiaceae, which is native in Southwest Asia. It grows in abundance in Thailand. There are several species of Kratom, each has their own qualities. We won't go into each one, but for illustrative purposes, I will name the different species of Kratom here:

- Maeng Da Kratom
- Bali Kratom
- Malaysian Kratom
- Borneo Kratom
- Thai Kratom
- Green Vein Kratom
- Indonesian Kratom

For hundreds, if not thousands of years, the Kratom leaves have been used an herbal "drug." It is often used in folk medicine and has very interesting properties. At low doses, it acts as a stimulant and at high doses, it is a powerful sedative. These qualities make it a perfect target for recreational use but also for medicinal use as well. It is a very powerful painkiller, Anti-diarrhea agent, and especially effective in the treatment of opiate addiction. Many people also swear by Kratom as an effective treatment for arthritis, restless legs syndrome (RLS), and fibromyalgia.

It is fairly long lasting in its effects, usually up to five hours. Like all things, it has side effects for some individuals; it can range from simple itchiness to seizures. Some people can become addicted to it if taken in excess. Although it is not itself an opiate, it acts like one and thus its ability to help with opiate withdrawal.

In the United States, 15 deaths have been reported that were supposedly linked to Kratom between 2014 and 2015. FAR less than those who die from Opiate addiction EVERYDAY! According to The American Society of Addiction Medicine or the ASAM, 18,893 people have died from overdoses on Opiate medications in 2014 ALONE. Another 10,574 have died from Heroin overdose in the same year.

(http://www.asam.org/docs/default-source/advocacy/opioid-addiction-disease-facts-figures.pdf)

In all fairness, some of these deaths may not have been directly attributed to Kratom since many of those who died were taking other substances **INADDITION** to Kratom, so it is difficult to directly link those deaths to Kratom alone. Even at 15 deaths, it is still much better than 18,893 deaths.

There are several ways to ingest Kratom, the most common are the following:

- **Powders** – stems and leaves ground into a powder form. This is the most popular version.
- **Leaves** – can be chewed
- **Tincture** – it can be turned into a tincture.
- **Extract** – this method increases its potency.
- **Capsules** – Due to its bitter taste, often people will put the powder into capsules.

There are many vendors online for the product and for the most part, most vendors sell authentic Kratom; it is growing in abundance, so there is no black market for it, at least not yet. In 2 weeks from the date of this writing, it will most definitely go underground, and then it will become dangerous and some vendors will sell bogus Kratom no doubt about it. In this next chapter, I want to discuss

Kratom as an alternative remedy for those going through Opioid addiction and withdrawal, for that is the real benefit of this herb. Sure, people will use it recreationally, but its true potential is lifesaving, and that is why this DEA ban is just ridiculous. We will discuss that in a future chapter.

Its Usefulness for Opioid Addiction And Withdrawal

The reason Kratom works so well for people who are addicted to opioids and Heroin is because its main ingredient, Mitragynine is an opioid agonist; Kratom also contains an alkaloid called 7-hyrdoxymitragynine which has been proven to be a very powerful opioid agonist as well. Meaning, it mimics the sedative and pain killing effects of drugs like Hydrocodone, Heroin, morphine and other related substances with far fewer Side effects.

Kratom is effective because it activates the supraspinal mu- and delta- opioid receptors; this is the reason why it helps those in withdrawal from opioids and Heroin. It is also the reason why so many use it as an alternative since it has an opioid-like effect upon the body. People have reported almost 100% relief from withdrawal symptoms while using Kratom.

In a study conducted By Christopher McCurdy of the school of Pharmacy at the University of Mississippi found the following results using Kratom for withdrawal symptoms.

"Mitragynine completely blocked all withdrawal symptoms and could provide a remarkable step-down-like

treatment for people addicted to hardcore narcotics such as morphine, oxycodone or Heroin,"

He goes on to add that many of the reports of people overdosing or dying from Kratom are, as I stated earlier due to mixing of other drugs with Kratom.

He states, **"We have been able to distinguish the effects of Kratom from those of other drugs whose presence was unanticipated," he said. "This has allowed us to document that some toxicity of Kratom is actually from other pharmaceutical agents that had been added."** (http://news.olemiss.edu/new-hope-for-addicts/#.UkSzEeg9-cc)

So many studies exist of the benefits of Kratom. Here is a list of links of interest.

- Total Synthesis of (-)-Mitragynine and Analogues
- Kratom Studied as Opiate Suppressor
- 53. MITRAGYNA Korthals, Observ. Naucl. Indic. 19. 1839, nom. cons.,
  not Mitragyne R. Brown (1810).
- Kratom and Other Mitragynines: The Chemistry and Pharmacology of Opiods from a Non-Opium Source
- Evaluation of Antioxidant and Antibacterial Activities of Aqueous, Methanolic and Alkaloid Extracts from Mitragyna
  Speciosa (Rubiaceae Family) Leaves

- Pharmacology of Kratom: An Emerging Botanical Agent With Stimulant, Analgesic and Opioid-Like Effects
- Antidepressant-like effect of mitragynine isolated from Mitragyna speciosa Korth in mice model of depression.
- Total Synthesis of (-)-Mitragynine and Analogues
- In-Utero Effects of the Crude Ethanolic Extract of the Leaves of Mitragyna speciosa on Neural Tube Formation in Rats

- Mitragyna speciosa Korth standardized methanol extract induced short-term potentiation of CA1 subfield in rat hippocampal slices

- Self-treatment of opioid withdrawal using Kratom (Mitragynia speciosa korth)
- Computational Study on the Conformations of Mitragynine and Mitragynaline
- Simultaneous analysis of mitragynine, 7-hydroxymitragynine, and other alkaloids in the psychotropic plant "Kratom" (Mitragyna speciosa) by LC-ESI-MS
- Pharmacology of Kratom: an emerging botanical agent with stimulant, analgesic and opioid-like effects.
- Neurosoup Kratom Page
- List of alkaloids identified in Mitragyna speciosa Kratom, and their known or potential activity
- Acute Toxicity Study of Standardized Mitragyna speciosa Korth Aqueous Extract in Sprague Dawley Rats

- Evaluation of the Effects of Mitragyna speciosa Alkaloid Extract on Cytochrome P450 Enzymes Using a High Throughput Assay
- Sedative, Cognitive Impairment and Anxiolytic Effects of Acute Mitragyna Speciosa in Rodents
- Ethnophrmacology of Kratom and the Mitragyna Alkaloids
- Acute and long-term effects of alkaloid extract of Mitragyna speciosa on food and water intake and body weight in rats.
- Pharmacological Studies on 7-Hydroxymitragynine, Isolated from the Thai Herbal Medicine Mitragyna speciosa:Discovery of an Orally Active Opioid Analgesic
- In Vitro and in Vivo Effects of Three Different Mitragyna speciosa Korth Leaf Extracts on Phase II Drug Metabolizing Enzymes—Glutathione Transferases (GSTs)
- The neuromuscular blockade produced by pure alkaloid, mitragynine and methanol extract of Kratom leaves (Mitragyna speciosa Korth.)
- Genes induced by high concentration of salicylic acid in Mitragyna speciosa

Why Is Kratom Being Banned?

Despite some of the risks that Kratom may pose to SOME individuals, its usefulness for drug addiction and recovery has been demonstrated by countless people. It seems like whenever the alternative health industry finds something that actually works the government, and the drug companies join together and try to ban it. This is exactly what is happening to Kratom as well.

On September 30th, 2016, Kratom will be classified as a schedule 1 drug, meaning it is in the same category as marijuana. According to the DEA, Kratom is dangerous. They base this on the fact that from 2010 to 2015 the U.S. Poison Control Centers have received 660 calls related to the Kratom herb. That is 132 calls a year and less than 1 call per day. However, calls regarding over the counter painkillers such as aspirin, Tylenol, etc. received 300,000 call in that same time frame. That is 60,000 a year and 164 calls PER DAY. However, Kratom is the one that is being banned. Yes, aspirin is far more accessible and that is partly to do with such high numbers, but Kratom is also widely used by thousands of people so 132 calls a year is an extremely low number. Just like those who did not use aspirin as intended, so too did those not use Kratom as intended and ended up being poisoned by it. Its common sense.

Here is the DEA in their own words:

Now here is an interesting little fact about the DEA's ban on Kratom. The DEA will ban it temporarily for up to three years so it can be "determined" whether it has any viable medical uses. In other words, when the pharmaceutical companies deem it fit for public consumption, which will most likely be never, **OR** until they can make it more powerful than the current drugs, they produce in the Opioid Sector.

I know this might sound like some grand conspiracy theory. I thought the same thing until I poked around a bit and found Big Pharma has quite an interest in Kratom. In fact, they are betting on both sides of the coin. On one side, they are researching to see if they can make money off Kratom and on the other side of the coin, they are lobbying the government to ban it. Why both sides? Its genius! They are hedging their bets. If it turns out to be useful, they will create their own Kratom-derived products and control its use. If they find that they can't make money on it, they will keep it banned so it won't compete with their existing opioid market. **It is sheer genius.** It is certainly not the first time they used this tactic.

Do you recall when marijuana was universally illegal in the United States? The pharmaceutical community and the government agencies were adamant that marijuana was dangerous. However, when big pharma was able to synthesis Marijuana or rather its active component THC, suddenly marijuana started to become legal and law enforcement started to reduce its penalties for those caught with it. For example, the drug Marinol, created the Solvay Pharmaceuticals Inc mimics THC. As big pharma found ways to make money off it, suddenly its legal status started to change. I think that is suspicious.

Let's take a quick look at big pharma's interest in Kratom. From 2008 to 2016, big pharma created 3 synthetic opioids derived from KRATOM. Yes, you read that correctly, DERIVED FROM KRATOM. These Synthetic Opioids are called MGM-9. MGM-15 and MGM-16.

The first study published in 2008 states:

"Mitragynine is a major indole alkaloid isolated from the Thai medicinal plant Mitragyna speciosa that has opium-like properties, although its chemical structure is quite different from that of morphine. We attempted to develop novel analgesics derived from mitragynine, and thus synthesized the ethylene glycol-bridged and C10-fluorinated derivative of mitragynine, MGM-9 [(E)-methyl 2-(3-ethyl-7a,12a-(epoxyethanoxy)-9-fluoro-1,2,3,4,6,7,12,12b-octahydro-8-methoxyindolo[2,3-a]quinolizin-2-yl)-3-methoxyacrylate]."

SOURCE: -
http://www.ncbi.nlm.nih.gov/pubmed/18550129

The Second Study, published as recently as 2014 states:

"In this study, we developed dual-acting μ- and δ-opioid agonists MGM-15 and MGM-16 from 7-hydroxymitragynine for the treatment of acute and chronic pain."

SOURCE: -
http://jpet.aspetjournals.org/content/348/3/383.full

The interesting phrase here is " ...*for the treatment of acute and chronic pain.*"

That statement makes it clear that they are actively working with Kratom to **MAKE A PRODUCT OF THEIR OWN.**

So now that Kratom is illegal, big pharma has no competition for their existing drugs AND they have plenty of time to develop products from Kratom and keep it under their control. Doesn't anyone see this as highly suspect?

There are also many patents on Kratoms alkaloids.

Go to http://patft.uspto.gov/netahtml/PTO/search-bool.html

Input these keywords In the Search:

Kratom

7-hydroxymitragynine

Mitragynine

You will notice so many of them. At first, some do not look relevant, but if you click on them and then search the page for one or all the keywords, you will find them.

The DEA's ban of a drug that killed maybe 15 people and let's says 7 of those overdosed on Kratom alone, is not reason enough for a ban. Meanwhile big pharma makes millions of opioid painkillers that kill thousands a year, and they say nothing. The government official stance is that people are not using the Opioids as intend and therefore, the drug companies should not be banned from making them. If we use that logic, there is no reason to ban Kratom just because a few people do not use it as intended.

Although there is no official body to regulate or distill Kratom doesn't make it any more dangerous than anything else. Big pharma simply can't control the market, and therefore, it wants it to be banned. They will now hijack Kratom, study it intently, and they will start to control its distribution once the opioid addiction issues hit a nadir. If Kratom stays legal who knows what would happen to big pharma's pain pill market? It won't disappear, but it will be dented.   When Marijuana was legalized in several states, Medication purchase and use went down dramatically.

According to Bradford and Bradford, Health Affairs, July 2016, when marijuana was made legal in several states, there was **1826 fewer doses** of pain medication. **These are Annual Drug doses prescribed _PER PHYSICIAN._** ---

http://content.healthaffairs.org/content/35/7/1230.abstract

In light of the above, there is clear evidence that the pharmaceuticals have had their eye on Kratom for quite some time now, and it is only now they, with government cooperation have decided to make it illegal for the average person. What is also suspicious is the timing, the opioid crisis is hitting its peak, its time for them to come up with safer options, Kratom has proven to be safer. So why not control it? Do you see what I mean?

A Boon For Others

Aside from big pharma, law enforcement is also against the legalization of marijuana for the same reason they are against keeping Kratom legal. With drugs being legal, arrests go down. That means the need for cops will diminish. In addition, the prison system which is largely a private business affair would lose money. It is so apparent that the banning of Kratom is just a way to make up for the legalization of Marijuana; they want to nip Kratom in the bud so to speak.

Another industry that is against the legalization of Kratom, and Marijuana has always been the Alcohol companies. An example of this is the campaign contributions the California Beer & Beverage Distributors made to a committee dedicated to preventing the legalization of marijuana. Why you say? Pure and simple, Marijuana and Kratom, for that matter, are competition to alcohol. The alcohol companies know full well that most people don't drink in moderation. People are drinking to get a buzz, Kratom and Marijuana provide superior effects and are therefore, a threat to the alcohol industry. It's ironic that an industry that was once prohibited is in favor of the prohibition of another substance. It's funny how that is.

On May 24th, 2016, in "Huddle," a daily Politico Newsletter for Government Insiders contained a paid advertisement from the "Wine And Spirits wholesalers of America." It is hilarious, at least to me it is. Here is the Ad text and judge for yourself.

" ** A message from Wine & Spirits Wholesalers of America: While neutral on the issue of legalization, WSWA believes states that legalize marijuana need to ensure appropriate and effective regulations are enacted to protect the public from the dangers associated with the abuse and misuse of marijuana.

23 states and the District of Columbia have legalized medicinal marijuana while Alaska, Colorado, Oregon, Washington and D.C. have legalized possession and recreational use. In the years since the state legalized medicinal use, Colorado law enforcement officials have documented a significant increase in traffic fatalities in which drivers tested positive for marijuana.

Congress should fully fund Section 4008 of the FAST Act (PL 114-94) in the FY 2017 Appropriations process to document the prevalence of marijuana impaired driving, outline impairment standards and determine driving impairment detection methods."

Read more at http://thefreethoughtproject.com/wikilieaks-marijuana-alcohol-lobby/#hegemAozCHD7ic84.99

This ad coming from an industry that is responsible for more traffic fatalities than any other. They seem highly concerned for "driver" safety due to marijuana consumption. They don't seem too concerned about their own role in any accidents. It smells like bullshit to me, or rather, it smells more like they are afraid they won't be the only drug pusher in town.

The Response To The Ban

As you may have surmised, there is quite an uproar over the ban of Kratom. A Petition was created and signed by 117,666 people urging the President to do something about the ban.
https://petitions.whitehouse.gov/petition/please-do-not-make-Kratom-schedule-i-substance

The number of signatures is significant. In order for the administration to take any request seriously, there needs to be at 100,000 signatures. They have received well above that. Unfortunately, it is doubtful the administration will do much of anything. Even so, they need to have a good justification as to why it should be banned as opposed to the scant evidence the DEA has brought forward. The Congress as well has not said a thing. Although the DEA has the right to impose a ban on substances, they feel might be dangerous to the public, the Congress has the ability to block that move by reducing funding. Again, this most likely will not happen since big pharma has a huge role in this ban. The most progressive of members in Congress have either declined to comment or have not even responded to attempts made for their stance on the ban.

Shops across the country are defying the ban. For example, the Dragon Herbarium in Portland is one of them. 50% of their total sales come from Kratom. This ban will force them to fire half their workers. They and many other shops selling Kratom are hoping against hope that the Ban is reversed. This ban is insane, and I suspect the fallout will be much more intense as September 30th arrives, the day Kratom is officially banned.

Final Thoughts

The ban on Kratom is insane; the DEA has no substantial evidence for it, and thus it makes the ban highly suspect. They should have left legalization up to the states. Some states have already banned Kratom but now all of them will have to.

In those states that Kratom is banned, we have already seen a spike in Opioid deaths. Alabama alone has seen a spike in Opioid deaths, a spike of 20% since Kratom was banned:

https://www.rt.com/usa/358931-Kratom-drug-dea-schedule/

We need Kratom to stay legal, the percentage of opioid addicts in certain areas is too high. Castlight Health did a study of Painkiller abuse across the country and found a staggering amount of abuse.

Chattanooga, TN: 7.7% of the population has developed an abuse issue.

Evansville-Henderson, IN: 7.8 % of the population.

Oklahoma City, OK: 4 out of 50 people abuse painkillers.

Odessa, TX: 8% of the population.

Hickory, NC: 9.9% of the population.

Panama City, FL: 11.5% of the population.

Wilmington, NC: 11.6%

Just to name a few. You can see the study results here:

http://healthversed.com/2016/07/20-most-drug-addicted-cities-in-america/

These numbers are staggering. We clearly need alternatives and Kratom was the best thus far.

If you want to have your voice heard, please sign the petition below, maybe for once the government will actually listen to the people and allow individuals to make their own decisions for a change. It is one thing if Kratom caused massive devastation, but it hasn't and therefore, a ban is unwarranted.

Come September 30th, mark my words, an increase in Opioid Overdoses and deaths will rise. I suppose time will tell.

Sign the petition:

https://petitions.whitehouse.gov/petition/please-do-not-make-Kratom-schedule-i-substance

Recommended Reading

Kratom : The Bible - From the Heavens: Quitting Pain Pills & Opiates with this Divine Leaf!

Kratom: Kratom for Beginners, Kratom Plants, Kratom Pills, Kratom Powders, Everything You Need to Know (Kratom, Kratom Books)

KRATOM: A Comprehensive Guide to Understanding the Effects and Benefits of this Amazing Plant: (and everything you want to know to get started with kratom).

Chasing the Scream: The First and Last Days of the War on Drugs

Current and Upcoming Books by the Author

www.simonluria.com

Current:

The Panama Papers: The Largest Financial Scandal of Modern Times

The NSA Hack and its Implications

Is Big Pharma Behind The Ban on Kratom?

Is Trump Clinton's Puppet?

UPCOMING:

The Self Victimization of A People: How Judaism Fosters Antisemitism

Outlaws of Islam: The Great Satan of the East

Krokodil Tears: The Drug That Could Destroy the World

The False Promise of Reward: How Society Promotes Addiction

Source Material

https://petitions.whitehouse.gov/petition/please-do-not-make-Kratom-schedule-i-substance

http://www.kens5.com/news/health/dea-to-make-Kratom-a-schedule-1-subtance-at-the-end-of-this-months/315385905

https://www.theodysseyonline.com/the-war-on-Kratom

https://www.statnews.com/2016/08/30/Kratom-ban-dea-schedule-1/

http://thefreethoughtproject.com/pharma-Kratom-dea-patent/

http://thefreethoughtproject.com/big-pharma-synthesizing-cannabis-patent-able-pill-killing-people/

https://www.washingtonpost.com/news/wonk/wp/2016/07/13/one-striking-chart-shows-why-pharma-companies-are-fighting-legal-marijuana/

http://content.healthaffairs.org/content/35/7/1230.abstract

http://www.marketwatch.com/story/how-the-dea-could-introduce-big-pharma-to-marijuana-2016-07-01

http://heavy.com/news/2016/09/dea-drug-enforcement-agency-ban-Kratom-deaths-opiates-Heroin-united-states-penalties-testimonials-poison-control-petition/

http://thefifthcolumnnews.com/2016/09/scheduling-of-Kratom-by-dea-protects-big-pharma/

http://personalliberty.com/police-department-points-to-big-pharma-as-major-dealer-in-drug-war/

http://personalliberty.com/police-department-points-to-big-pharma-as-major-dealer-in-drug-war/

https://www.leafly.com/news/politics/the-top-5-industries-lobbying-against-cannabis-legalization-will/

http://www.huffingtonpost.com/entry/petition-Kratom-ban-dea_us_57d051e7e4b06a74c9f2177a

http://www.kptv.com/story/33044135/portland-shop-challenges-deas-move-to-make-Kratom-illegal

https://www.theguardian.com/us-news/2016/sep/11/Kratom-federal-crackdown-backlash-opioid-addiction

http://www.fosters.com/news/20160908/banning-Kratom-is-wrong-policy

http://www.huffingtonpost.com/entry/congress-Kratom-ban-dea_us_57d1ad7ce4b03d2d45993e0e

http://thelibertarianrepublic.com/white-house-will-justify-Kratom-ban/

http://www.philosophers-stone.co.uk/?p=14168

https://www.rt.com/usa/358931-Kratom-drug-dea-schedule/

About The Author

Simon Luria is a writer, raised in London and now based out of New York City. Far from flying under the radar, his name is often enough to start heated debates. On the one side, his fans adore him, always with their eye on his next book. On the other side, there is a vocal group of people who loathe Simon. These people vehemently oppose everything that he says, protesting him at every turn.

For his part, Simon makes no effort to quell this distaste, never seeking out controversy but at the same time never taking any steps to avoid it either. He lets the chips fall where they may. He sees the modern world as unnecessarily sanitized and politically correct, Simon refuses to fold under pressure, sticking to his principles, always telling it like he sees it. He is known for delivering blunt, well-researched musings on finance, geopolitics, foreign policy, religion, medicine, and the state of the world. His opinions have caused him to shield his true identity. It's the only way for him to produce the work he does without fear.

www.simonluria.com

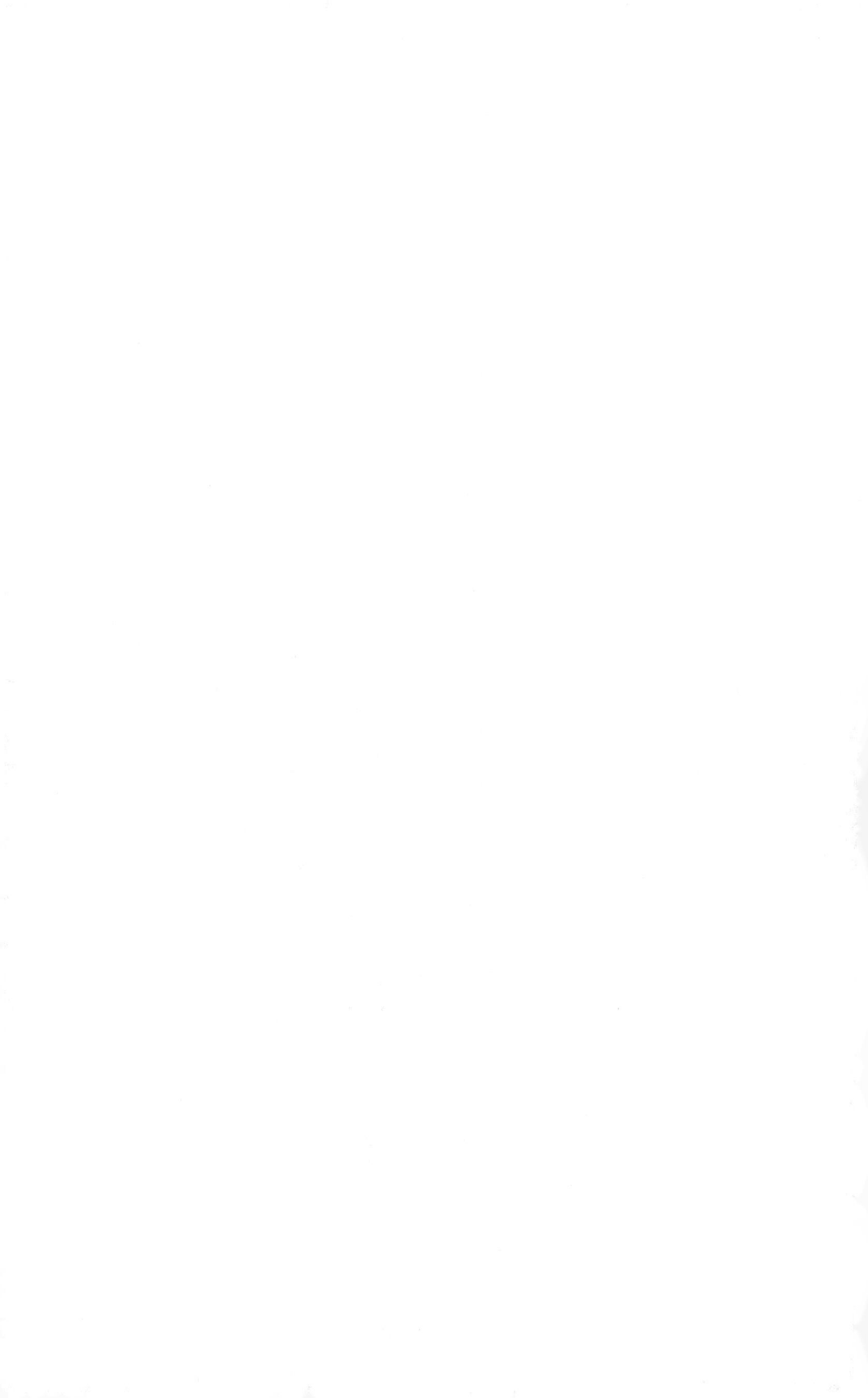

www.ingramcontent.com/pod-product-compliance
Lightning Source LLC
Chambersburg PA
CBHW070250290526
45789CB00004B/1817